Low Fodmap Diet Cookbook

Table of Contents

SNACKS --5

Wontons (Dumplings) --5

Veggie Burgers--8

Savory Muffin --- 10

Tzatziki Dip-- 13

Spiced Molasses Cookies -- 15

Vegetable Muffins -- 17

Peanut Butter Energy Bars --- 19

Pumpkin hummus -- 21

Kale Chips --- 23

Turkey, Brie & Cranberry Filo Pastries------------------------------------- 25

Pumpkin & Zucchini Savoury Slice -- 27

Roasted Polenta Bites with Cheese & Herbs--------------------------- 29

50 VEGETARIAN RECIPES --- 32

Low FODMAP Yellow Snack Cake with Rainbow Sprinkles--------------------------- 32

Low FODMAP Coconut Lime Bread --- 34

Low FODMAP Smoked Gouda Apple Muffins -------------------------------- 36

Low FODMAP Beer Bread --- 39

Low FODMAP Hazelnut Shortcake with   Berries & Caramel -----41

Low FODMAP Fluffy Pancakes --44

LOW FODMAP SUN-DRIED TOMATO PESTO --- 46

LOW FODMAP MASALA CHAI -- 48

VEGAN LOW FODMAP CRISP TOPPING--- 50

LOW FODMAP PEACHES AND CREAM POPSICLES WITH RASPBERRIES ------------ 52

LOW FODMAP NO-CHURN VANILLA ICE CREAM WITH CHOCOLATE COVERED ALMONDS --- 54

LOW FODMAP NO-CHURN VANILLA ICE CREAM -- 56

LOW FODMAP CANTALOUPE, CUCUMBER AND BURRATA SALAD ------------------- 58

LOW FODMAP CARROT-GINGER SOUP --- 60

LOW FODMAP TOFU SALAD --- 62

LOW FODMAP ORANGE CARROT JUICE -- 64

LOW FODMAP CREAM OF TOMATO SOUP WITH GRILLED CHEESE CROUTONS- 66

LOW FODMAP CARAMELIZED PINEAPPLE SAUCE --------------------------------------- 68

LOW FODMAP RANCH DRESSING --- 70

LOW FODMAP PASTA PRIMAVERA --- 72

LOW FODMAP GRATED CARROT SALAD --- 74

NO FODMAP FRUIT SALAD -- 76

NO FODMAP MALT VINEGAR SALAD DRESSING --------------------------------------- 77

NO FODMAP VEGETABLE SALAD -- 79

LOW FODMAP EGGPLANT DIP -- 80

LOW FODMAP CARROT CONSOMMÉ --- 82

EASY STOVETOP LOW FODMAP MAC AND CHEESE------------------------------------ 84

LOW FODMAP JAPANESE PICKLES -- 86

LOW FODMAP LEMON GRANITA---**88**

Snacks

Wontons (Dumplings)

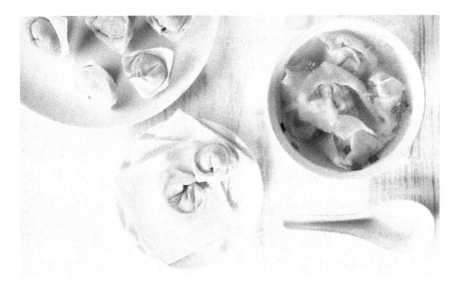

Time duration- 1 hour

Serving time: 60 wontons

Ingredients

Pork, lean, minced (maybe a combination of prawns, chicken, or even beef)

1 Tablespoon of cornstarch

Sesame oil for 2 tsp

3 teaspoons of ginger, grated

1/2 cup of green onion tops for spring, very finely chopped

2 Tbsp (to taste) soy sauce

1 cup of common or red cabbage, very finely diced

1 Tbsp of rice flour or tapioca

60 Wonton Square Wrappers

Preparation Method

- To make the wonton filling, consolidate the mince, cornstarch, sesame oil, ginger, green spring onion tops, soy sauce, and cabbage in a huge blending bowl. Cover and refrigerate until prepared to utilize.

- Gently dust a preparing plate secured with non-leave paper with rice or custard flour. To make wontons, place a chunk of 2 teaspoons of filling in the middle, brush 2 right point edges with water, and overlap on the askew creation sure any air is removed while fixing. Spot the completed wonton on the preparing sheet ensuring they don't contact one another. This corner to corner overlap is a straightforward one yet you can without much of a stretch overlay into various shapes.

- For bubbled wontons:

- Heat an enormous pot of water. When bubbling, add the wontons and cook for 5-6 minutes until the coast. Eliminate and channel in a softly oiled colander ensuring they are somewhat oiled all finished so they don't stay together.

- For sautéed wontons:
- Warmth a little unbiased oil in a skillet and fry wontons until the bottoms are earthy colored. Add some bubbling water and spread the dish with a tight-fitting cover. Steam-fry wontons for around 5 minutes or until cooked through.

Nutritional Value

1336 Kj / 319 cal Energy

The 21.80 g Protein

40.40 g Carbohydrates

1.30 g sugar

8.40 g Total Fat

2.60 g of Saturated Fat

2.00 g Fibre

Veggie Burgers

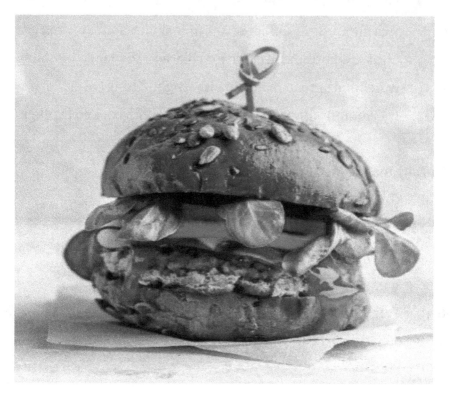

Time Duration- 1 hour 30 minutes

Serves: 8

Ingredients

Mashed fried potato

1/2 cup of rice which is cooked

Bread crumbs that are gluten-free

1 medium, grated carrot

1/2 thin, grated zucchini

2 Tbsp parmesan shaved cheese (optional)

2 Tbsp of new parsley from the continent

1 Tbsp of fresh cilantro

Grated Ginger

1 single egg

1 Tbsp of (gluten-free) soy sauce

Preparation Method

- Strip and steam potatoes until extremely delicate. Crush potato and leave aside or spot in the ice chest to chill off.
- Bubble/steam rice and permit to (cool in the cooler for quicker outcomes).
- Wash and finely hack new coriander and parsley.
- Mesh carrot and zucchini and eliminate any overabundance of fluid.
- When potato and rice have chilled off, place into a bowl with all fixings.
- Fold burgers into balls.
- Splash or sprinkle olive oil into a container or on a BBQ plate. Warmth oiled skillet/BBQ plate first before setting burgers.
- When burgers are in the container/on BBQ plate, permit them to cook for around 5 minutes before tenderly leveling burgers marginally.
- Cook burgers on low-medium warmth for roughly 15 minutes and just turn them once.

Nutritional Value

596 Kj / 142 cal Energy

5.60 g protein

15.80 g Carbohydrates

3.80 g Sugar

5.80 g Total Fat

2.30 g of Saturated Fat

2.40 g Fibre

Savory Muffin

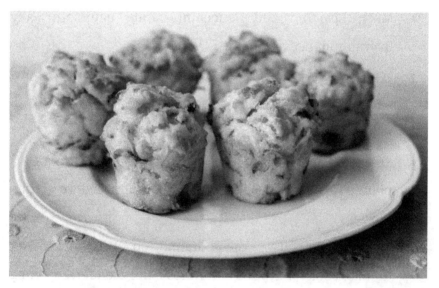

Time Duration- 25 minutes

Servings: 12

Ingredients

1 1/4 cup flour with tapioca

1 ¼ cup maize flour

Baking Powder 51/4 tsp

xanthan gum 13/4 tsp

3/4 cup of oat bran

Three Eggs

3/4 cup of cream

3/4 cup milk, low fat, milk-free from lactose

1 cup of crumbled feta cheese

1 cup of capsicum, red, beautifully diced

3/4 cup leaves of basil (roughly chopped)

Grated cheese for each muffin on top

To top each muffin, paprika

Preparation Method

- Preheat stove to 160°C/320°F and on a lower rack of the broiler, half fill a preparing plate with bubbling water (see tip beneath).
- Filter flour, preparing powder and thickened into a huge bowl, at that point add the grain (blend once more).
- In a different bowl, whisk eggs with the cream and milk.
- Add capsicum, disintegrated feta, and basil to the egg blend.
- Make a well in the flour blend and overlay wet blend into the dry fixings (you may need to add more milk to accomplish a somewhat messy batter, however not very wet).

- Spot huge biscuit cases in a biscuit plate and splash well with canola oil.
- Fill biscuit cases (see tip underneath) and tap down the top surface with a wet finger.
- Sprinkle the highest point of every biscuit with ground cheddar, at that point paprika.
- Prepare for around 17 minutes until brilliant earthy colored (an embedded stick ought to be perfect when taken out).
- Cool in the plate for 5 minutes, at that point put on a wire rack to cool further.

Nutritional Value

1104 Kj / 264 Cal of Energy

5.40 g protein

36.00 g Carbohydrates

2.70 g Sugar

10.80 g Total Fat

6.80 g of Saturated Fat

1.30 g Fibre

Tzatziki Dip

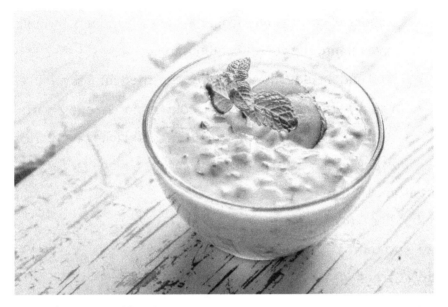

Time duration- 10 minutes

Serves: 50

Ingredients

Simple Greek yogurt (free with lactose if required)

3 cucumbers, sliced thinly

2 cloves of garlic, sliced in half

11/2 tsp of olive oil

1 Tbsp dried flakes of mint

Preparation Method

- Add garlic cloves to olive oil and leave to the side for a couple of moments to inject into the oil.
- Void yogurt into an enormous bowl.

- Blend through cucumber (dispose of fluid that originates from slashing the cucumber) and mint.
- Dispose of garlic cloves from the olive oil and mix through olive oil into the yogurt combination.
- Trial and include more cucumber or dried mint if you like.
- A spot in the cooler and serve cold in more modest parts: fill in as a plunge, with meat, in sandwiches, with rice dishes, cook potatoes, or in any case you like.

Nutritional Value

96 Kj / 23 cal of energy

1.20 g protein

1.10 g Carbohydrates

1.70 g sugar

1.40 g Total Fat

0.60 g of Saturated Fat

0.10 g Fibre

Spiced Molasses Cookies

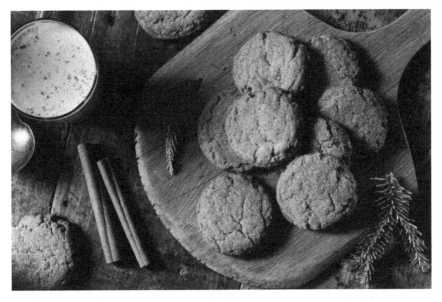

Time duration- 1 hour 20 minutes

Serving: 30

Ingredients

3/4 cup margarine or butter, melted

1 cup of sugar white

1 single egg

1/4 cup of molasses

2 cups white flour free of gluten

2 tsp powder for baking

1/2 tsp salt

1 Tsp of Cinnamon Ground

1/2 tsp nutmeg field

1/2 TL of ground ginger

Preparation Method

- In a huge bowl, join softened margarine, sugar, and egg and blend until smooth. Mix in molasses, flour, heating powder, salt, cinnamon, and all zest and mix until blend joins into a batter. Cover batter with saran wrap and refrigerate for in any event 60 minutes, or until mixture is firm.

- In the interim, preheat the broiler to 180°C/356°F and line an enormous heating plate with preparing the paper.

- Gap batter into 30 pecans measured pieces and fold into balls. Spot batter balls on the preparing plate ~5cm separated. Try not to smooth batter - treats will spread out as they heat.

- Heat treats in the stove for ~10 minutes, or until the highest points of treats start to break. Leave treats on a plate to cool marginally before moving onto a cooling stand.

Nutritional Value

478 Kj / 114 cal of Energy

The 0.40 g protein

17.00 g Carbohydrates

9.10 g Sugar

5.10 g Total Fat

1.00 g Saturated Fat

0.10 g Fibre

Vegetable Muffins

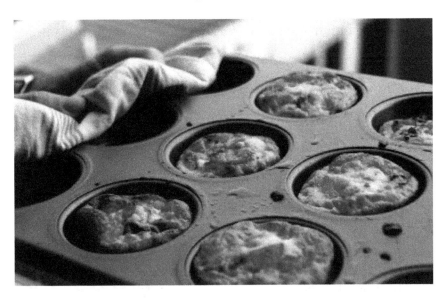

Time Duration- 45 minutes

Servings: 12

Ingredients

1 Capsicum in Red

Two tomatoes

1 bunch of chopped basil leaves

1 bunch of onions for the season, green tops only

Ten Eggs

1/2 cup of hard, grated cheese (e.g. cheddar)

1/2 tsp salt

Preparation Method

- Preheat broiler to 180°C/356°F.

- The flush external shell of eggs, break into an enormous bowl and whisk Chop the capsicum, tomatoes, basil, and spring onion and blend into the whisked eggs. Add salt.
- Mesh cheddar and put in a safe spot.
- Shower biscuit container with a non-stick splash. Empty blends into the biscuit plate.
- Sprinkle biscuits with cheddar.
- Spot plate in the broiler for 25-30 minutes.

Nutritional Value

376 Kj / 90 cal of Energy

7.50 g protein

2.60 g Carbohydrates

2.80 g Sugar

5.80 g Total Fat

2.80 g of Saturated Fat

0.60 g Fibre

Peanut Butter Energy Bars

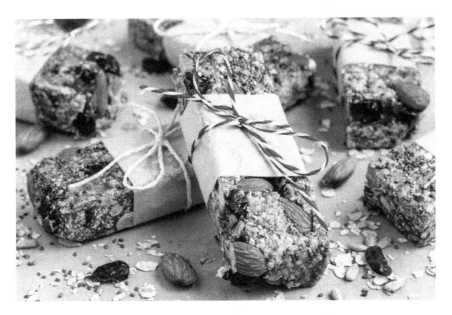

Serves: 12:

Time duration- 1 hour 10 minutes

Ingredients

1/2 cup of natural peanut butter (no sugar or salt added)

1/2 cup of sugar with maple

1 cup of rolled oats, toasted lightly,

1/2 cup of brown rice puffed in

1/2 cup flakes of quinoa

1/2 cup of thinly toasted almonds, chopped

1/4 cup dried, chopped cranberries

1/4 of a dried banana cup, chopped

1 Tbsp flakes of coconut, finely toasted

1 Tablespoon of Chia Seeds

1 Tbsp seeds of sunflower

Preparation Method

- Splash a 20cm x 20cm cut plate with cooking shower and line with preparing paper saved.

- In a little pan, heat nutty spread and maple syrup over low warmth, mixing until all-around joined.

- In a huge bowl, join dry fixings. Pour nut and maple syrup combination over dry fixings and mix until all-around joined.

- Move blend into the arranged plate, pushing down with marginally wet hands to guarantee combination is level and firmly pressed together.

- Refrigerate for in any event 1 hour before delicately eliminating from the plate and cutting into bars.

Nutritional Value

Power 907 Kj / 217 Cal

The 6.30 g protein

19.50 g Carbohydrates

5.60 g Sugar

12.30 g Total Fat

2.30 g of Saturated Fat

3.60 g Fibre

Pumpkin hummus

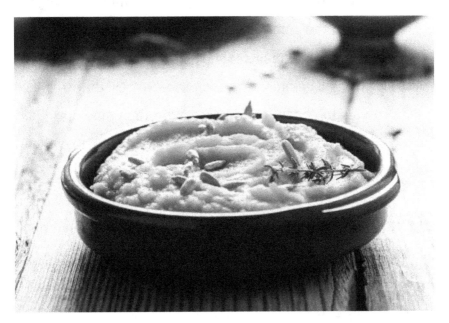

Serves: 3-4

Time duration- 35 mintes

Ingredients

Pumpkin from Kent / Jarrahdale, peeled and cut into 2 cm cubes

Two-tbs of tahini

2 tbs. olive oil filled with garlic

1 teaspoon cumin

1 tablespoon of Greek or natural yogurt

1 tablespoon lemon juice

1 Tsp of salt from the sea

Preparation Method

- Spot the pumpkin in a medium measured pot over medium warmth, with 2 tbs water and salt, and cover with a top.

Cook for 15-20 mins, mixing like clockwork. Add additional water in if the pumpkin resembles it's drying out. When the pumpkin is extra delicate, permit to cool.

- When the pumpkin has cooled, place pumpkin, tahini, salt, olive oil, and cumin into a food processor. On the off chance that you don't have a food processor, the pumpkin should be delicate enough to blend in with a fork/whisk. Blend until the consistency is smooth.

- Take out the pumpkin blend and fill the serving bowl. Mix through yogurt. Add additional salt or pepper, to your ideal taste.

Nutritional Value

Power 922 Kj / 220 Cal

3.20 g protein

8.10 g Carbohydrates

7.90 g Sugar

18.00 g Total Fat

Saturated Fat 2.60 g

4.6g Fibre

Kale Chips

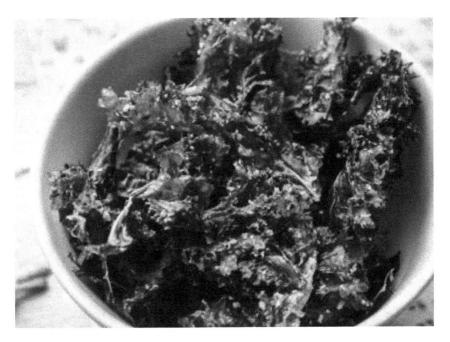

Servings: 4

Time duration- 20 minutes

Ingredients

1 handful of kale

1 Tablespoon of olive oil

2 Tbsp of pecorino cheese, finely grated cheese

The salt and pepper of the sea, to season

Preparation Method

- Preheat the broiler to 160°C/320°F.
- Line 2 heating plate with preparing paper.

- Eliminate the kale leaves from the stems and attack reduced down pieces. Wash kale pieces and dry.
- Join kale pieces, olive oil, and pecorino cheddar in a huge bowl.
- Spot kale onto the heating plate and prepare for 10-15 minutes or until leaves are fresh. Season with salt and pepper.

Nutritional Value

Power 283 Kj / 68 cal

2.20 g protein

1.50 g Carbohydrates

1.50 g sugar

5.70 g Total Fat

1.40 g Saturated Fat

1.50 g Fibre

Turkey, Brie & Cranberry Filo Pastries

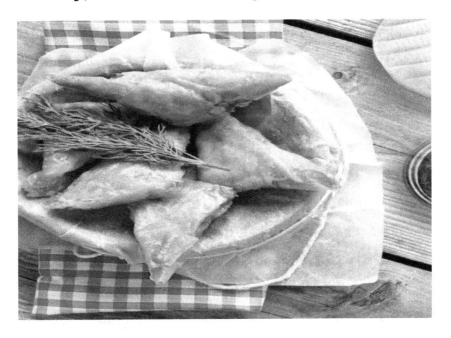

Time duration- 30 minutes

Servings: 10

Ingredients

13/4 cups of turkey fried, skinless, finely chopped

Brie cheese, sliced into little cubes

6 Tbsp cranberry sauce

41/2 Tbsp (recipe below) mayonnaise

3/4 cup chives, thinly chopped

3/4 cup of walnuts roasted, finely chopped

10 Sheets of Pastry Filo

Olive Spray Oil

Preparation Method

- Preheat broiler to 180°C/356°F.
- Blend the turkey, cheddar, cranberry sauce, chives, and mayonnaise in a bowl, season to taste with salt and pepper.
- Line a level heating sheet with non-stick paper and splash gently with olive oil.
- Cut filo sheets in equal parts the long way and cover with a somewhat sodden teatowel. On a level, workbench spread out one elliptical, splash the edges with olive oil, place the filling (40g) at the base, and crease consistently into triangles. Spot on the plate and shower the top with olive oil. Rehash until all the filling is utilized.
- Heat in the stove for 15-20 minutes until brilliant. Quickly slide onto permeable paper to retain overabundance oil and serve hot or warm.

Nutritional Value

1130 Kj / 270 Cal of Energy

The 15.90 g Protein

18.60 g Carbohydrates

5.20 g Sugar

14.50 g Total Fat

4.40 g of Saturated Fat

1.50 g Fibre

Pumpkin & Zucchini Savoury Slice

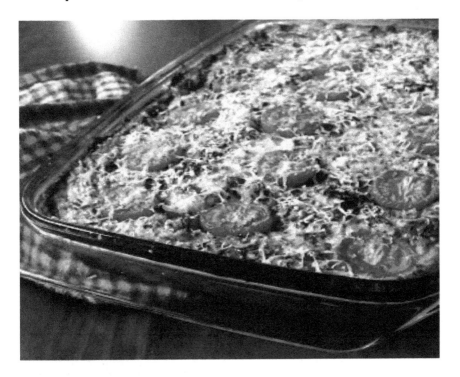

Time duration- I hour 10 minutes

Serves: 6

Ingredients

2 tsp of olive oil infused with garlic

Pumpkin, Japanese, grated

Five eggs

2 whites for eggs

1/4 cup of plain flour without gluten

1/2 cup of fat-reduced ricotta

Zucchini, grated, humidity removed

2 Teaspoons of fresh chives, chopped

2 Tbsp of fresh, chopped continental parsley

1/2 bunch of spring onions, just green tops

Cherry tomatoes from Punnet halved

1/2 cup delicious reduced-fat cheese, rubbed

Glaze balsamic, to serve

Preparation Method

- Preheat broiler to 180°C/356°F. Oil and line a 26x16cm (base estimation) cut skillet.

- Warmth oil in an enormous griddle. Cook ground pumpkin for 3-4 minutes or until starting to mollify.

- Whisk the eggs, egg whites, and flour in an enormous blending bowl until joined. Mix in ricotta, cooked pumpkin, zucchini, chives, parsley, and spring onion tips.

- Empty combination into the arranged cut container. Dissipate cherry tomatoes on top of blend and softly push down.

- Heat for 50 minutes or until gently brown and cooked through when tried with a stick.

- Sprinkle with ground cheddar and heat for a further 10 minutes, or until cheddar is liquefied and brilliant.

- Cut into 6 even pieces. Sprinkle with a balsamic coating to serve.

Nutritional Value

505 Kj / 121 cal of Energy

7.60 g protein

7.80 g Carbohydrates

2.70 g Sugar

6.20 g Total Fat

2.70 g of Saturated Fat

1.70 g fiber

Roasted Polenta Bites with Cheese & Herbs

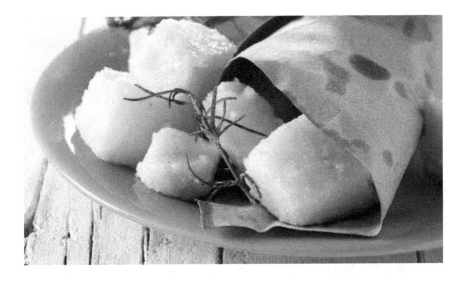

Time duration- 4 hours 30 minutes

Serves: 4

Ingredients

1 cup of polenta

1/2 cup of hard, grated cheese, e.g. Pecorino

1 Tbsp of new rosemary, finely chopped

Olive Spray Oil

Preparation Method

- Softly oil and line a 20 cm x 20 cm heating plate.
- Cook polenta as indicated by parcel directions (use water or low FODMAP stock in suggested amount).
- At the point when polenta has arrived at a smooth and thick consistency, add the cheddar and spices and mix to join. Eliminate from the heat at that point immediately fill an arranged plate. Tenderly tap and smooth surface with a spatula to straighten. Cover the surface with either plastic wrap or a sheet of preparing paper and permit to totally cool and set (~ 4 hours in the cooler, yet it is best left for the time being).
- At the point when set, rearrange polenta onto a hacking board and cut into the wanted shape (scaled-down triangles or square shapes function admirably).
- Preheat broiler to 240°C/464°F. Line a level preparing plate with non-leave paper and shower with olive oil. Spot nibbles on the plate guaranteeing they are isolated and neuter with olive oil. Cook for 20 minutes or until brilliant.
- Serve hot with some extra ground cheddar and spices dispersed over the top.

Nutritional Value

99 Kj / 24 cal of energy

1.90 g protein

1.80 g Carbohydrates

2.50 g Sugar

5.70 g Total Fat

1.30 g Saturated Fat

1.30 g Fibre

50 Vegetarian Recipes

Low FODMAP Yellow Snack Cake with Rainbow Sprinkles

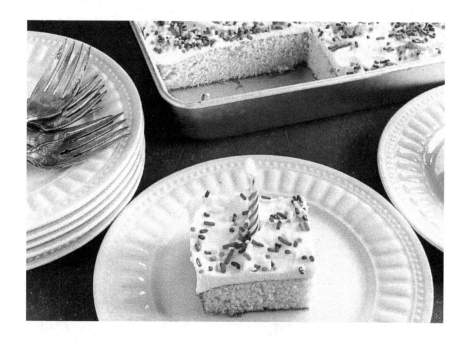

Makes: 24 Servings Prep Time: 10 minutes Total Time: 10 minutes

INGREDIENTS:

1 recipe Yellow Cake, baked in a 13-inch by 9-inch (33 cm by 23 cm) pan and cooled

1 batch Swiss Meringue Buttercream, freshly made and ready to use

Sprinkles; optional

Birthday candles; optional

PREPARATION:

Take out the cake from the pan. Frost your cake with buttercream. Sprinkle different sprinkles over your cake. Let it set and your cake is ready to serve.

If you are traveling somewhere with your cake then you do not need to take out a cake from the pan. Just decorate it in the pan and take it with you.

NUTRITION

Calories: 391kcal | Carbohydrates: 42g | Protein: 3g | Fat: 24g

Low FODMAP Coconut Lime Bread

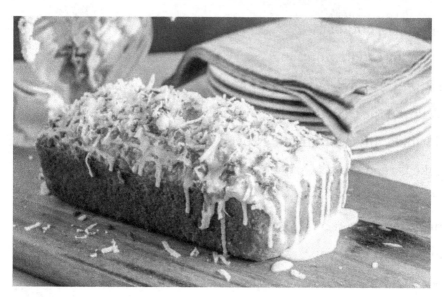

Makes: 12 Servings Prep Time: 10 minutes Cook Time: 1 hour

Total Time: 1 hour 10 minutes

INGREDIENTS:

Bread:

1 1/3 cups (194 g) low FODMAP gluten-free all-purpose flour, such as Bob's Red Mill 1 to 1 Gluten-Free Baking Flour

1 cup (198 g) sugar

1 teaspoon baking powder; use gluten-free if following a gluten-free diet

½ teaspoon salt

¾ cup (180 ml) canned full-fat coconut milk, at room temperature

½ cup (120 ml) unrefined coconut oil, melted and cooled

2 large eggs

2 tablespoons very fine lime zest, made with a rasp-style zester

1 tablespoon freshly squeezed lime juice

1 teaspoon vanilla extract

½ cup (38 g) plus 2 tablespoons sweetened flaked coconut, divided

Glaze & Topping:

1 cup (90 g) sifted confectioner's sugar

2 tablespoons freshly squeezed lime juice

2 tablespoons sweetened flaked coconut

1 tablespoon very fine lime zest, made with a rasp-style zester

PREPARATION:

For the bread:

Pre-heat your oven at 350°F (180°C). Line 8 ½-inch by 4 ¼-inch pan with parchment paper. Overhang the two sides and coat the paper and set aside.

Mix the flour, sugar, baking powder, and salt. Make a well in the center. In a separate bowl place the coconut milk, coconut oil, eggs, lime zest and juice, and vanilla extract and whisk together well.

Mix wet ingredients to dry ingredients and fold well. After it's done put the mixture in a pan. Place the loaf pan in the oven to bake the bread. Bake for at least 30 minutes. When it's done take it out and decorate with topping.

For topping:

Mix sugar and lime juice well together. Drizzle this glaze over cool bread. Let it set and then sprinkle lemon zest over it. The bread is ready to serve.

NUTRITION

Calories: 328kcal | Carbohydrates: 48g | Protein: 2g | Fat: 15g | Saturated Fat: 3g | Cholesterol: 3mg | Sodium: 172mg | Potassium: 44mg | Fiber: 2g | Sugar: 32g | Calcium: 1mg | Iron: 1mm

Low FODMAP Smoked Gouda Apple Muffins

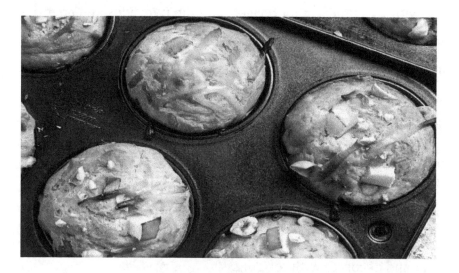

Makes: 12 Servings Prep Time: 10 minutes Cook Time: 15 minutes Total Time: 25 minutes

INGREDIENTS:

1 cup (240 ml) lactose-free whole milk, at room temperature

1 tablespoon lemon juice

2 cups (290 g) low FODMAP gluten-free all-purpose flour, such as Bob's Red Mill 1 to 1 Gluten-Free Baking Flour

1 ½ teaspoon baking powder; use gluten-free if following a gluten-free diet

½ teaspoon baking soda

¼ teaspoon salt

3 large eggs, at room temperature

½ cup (107 g) firmly packed light brown sugar

1/3 cup (75 ml) extra-virgin olive oil

1 medium-sized Pink Lady apple cored and diced (leave the peel on)

½ cup (50 g) chopped toasted, skinned hazelnuts

5- ounces (140 g) smoked gouda, shredded

PREPARATION:

Position rack in center of oven. Preheat oven to 425°F (220°C). Line 12 muffin cups with paper liners or coat with nonstick spray.

Mix lemon juice and milk well and set them aside to thicken. It takes around 5 minutes.

Besides mix flour, baking soda, baking powder, and salt in a large bowl. Make a well in a center and place it aside.

Beat brown sugar and eggs along with prepared sour milk and olive oil. Beat this mixture until it gets smooth.

Combine the dry ingredients with the wet mixture. Fold it well and add nuts, apple, and cheese. Put this mixture in a muffins tray to bake.

Bake muffins for 12 to 15 minutes or until you press a toothpick and it comes out clean. After getting done take them out and serve.

NUTRITION

Calories: 301kcal | Carbohydrates: 33g | Protein: 7g | Fat: 16g | Saturated Fat: 1g | Sodium: 226mg | Potassium: 16mg | Fiber: 1g | Sugar: 11g | Vitamin A: 8IU | Vitamin C: 1mg | Calcium: 1mg | Iron: 1mg

Low FODMAP Beer Bread

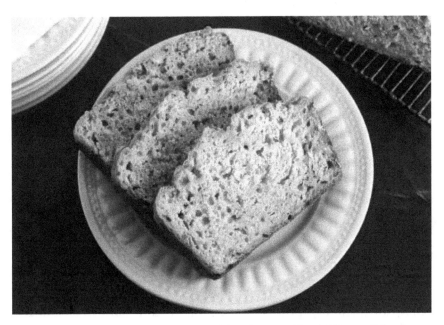

Makes: 12 Servings Prep Time: 10 minutes Cook Time: 50 minutes
Total Time: 1 hour

INGREDIENTS:

2 ½ cups (363 g) low FODMAP gluten-free all-purpose flour, such as Bob's Red Mill 1 to 1 Gluten-Free Baking Flour

½ cup (50 g) old-fashioned rolled oats; use gluten-free if following a gluten-free diet

1 tablespoon baking powder; use gluten-free if following a gluten-free diet

1 tablespoon sugar

1 teaspoon caraway seeds; optional

1 teaspoon salt

3 large eggs, at room temperature

3 tablespoons honey

3 tablespoons extra-virgin olive oil

12- ounce (360 ml) bottle or can of beer; use gluten-free if following a gluten-free diet

¼ cup (16 g) chopped scallions, green parts only; optional

½ cup (55 g) shredded cheddar cheese; divided and optional (I like sharp orange-colored cheddar)

PREPARATION:

Position rack in the middle of the oven. Preheat oven to 375°F (190°C). Coat a 9-inch by 5-inch (23 cm by 12 cm) loaf pan with nonstick spray, line the bottom with parchment paper allowing it to overhand the two short ends, then coat paper.

Whisk flour, baking powder, oats, sugar, and salt well in a big mixing bowl.

In other bowl mix eggs, honey and oil. Whisk this mixture well and add it to dry ingredients. Fold all mixture well until a smooth mixture is formed. After this add beer and fold again the mixture. Put the pan in the oven and bake it for 20 minutes. Take out and sprinkle cheese and again bake for 20 minutes or until the top gets golden brown. Take out the pan and let it cool. Take out the bread from the pan and serve.

NUTRITION

Calories: 267kcal | Carbohydrates: 40g | Protein: 6g | Fat: 7g | Saturated Fat: 1g | Sodium: 327mg | Potassium: 36mg | Fiber: 2g | Sugar: 5g | Calcium: 6mg | Iron: 1mg

Low FODMAP Hazelnut Shortcake with Berries & Caramel

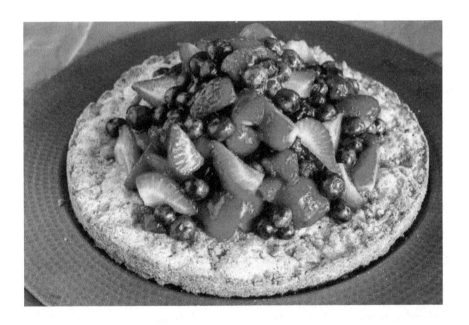

Makes: 8 Servings Prep Time: 20 minutes Cook Time: 30 minutes
Total Time: 50 minutes

INGREDIENTS:

Hazelnut Shortcake:

2- ounces (55 g) skinned, toasted hazelnuts

1 2/3 cups (241 g) low FODMAP gluten-free all-purpose flour, such as Bob's Red Mill 1 to 1 Baking Flour

¼ cup (54 g) plus 1 tablespoon firmly packed light brown sugar, divided

1 tablespoon baking powder; use gluten-free if following a gluten-free diet

½ teaspoon salt

1 cup (240 ml) lactose-free heavy cream

Berry Topping:

10- ounces (280 g) fresh strawberries, hulled and halved or quartered (depending on size), at room temperature

6- ounces (170 g) fresh blueberries, at room temperature

3- ounces (85 g) fresh raspberries, at room temperature

2- ounces (55 g) fresh blackberries, at room temperature

½ cup (120 ml) Low FODMAP Salted Caramel Sauce, fluid and ready to use

PREPARATION:

For the Shortcake: Position rack in the middle of the oven. Preheat oven to 400°F (200°C). Coat the inside of a 9-inch (23 cm) round springform pan with nonstick spray; set aside.

Grind nuts in the food processor by turning the button on and off. Put it in a bowl and add flour, baking powder, brown sugar, and salt. Mix all these ingredients well. Pour cream and mix well until a soft dough is formed.

Place this dough on a baking tray with fingers. Add remaining brown sugar on the top and bake it for 30 minutes. When it's done take it out and place it on the rack and cool down.

For the Filling & Assembly: Place all of the berries in a mixing bowl. Pour caramel sauce over the berries and fold gently, then mound on top of the shortcake. Serve immediately, cut into wedges.

NUTRITION

Calories: 386kcal | Carbohydrates: 54g | Protein: 4g | Fat: 14g | Sodium: 277mg | Fiber: 2g | Sugar: 9g

Low FODMAP Fluffy Pancakes

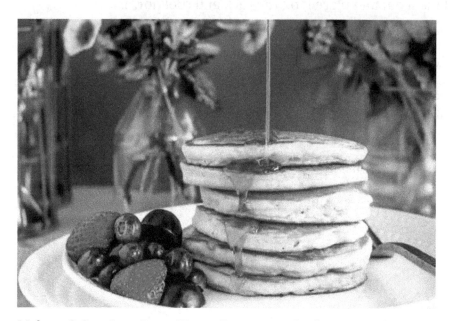

Makes: 8 Servings Prep Time: 5 minutes Cook Time: 15 minutes
Total Time: 20 minutes

INGREDIENTS:

2 cups (290 g) low FODMAP, gluten-free all-purpose flour, such as
Bob's Red Mill 1 to 1 Gluten-Free Baking Flour

¼ cup (50 g) sugar

1 tablespoon plus 1 teaspoon baking powder; use gluten-free if
following a gluten-free diet

½ teaspoon salt

¼ teaspoon baking soda

1 ¾ cups (420 ml) whole lactose-free milk, at room temperature

¼ cup (57 g; ½ stick) melted unsalted butter, cooled to just warm

1 large egg, at room temperature

1 teaspoon vanilla extract

PREPARATION:

Stir flour, baking powder, sugar, salt, and baking soda in a large bowl. Mix the wet ingredients in a separate bowl.

Mix all of the wet mixtures into dry ingredients and fold well.

Place a non-stick pan overheat. Spread the batter on the pan and cook on medium heat. Cook it until bubbles are formed and the bottom gets golden brown. Turn it and cook from another side as well. Serve it with hot maple syrup.

NUTRITION

Calories: 253kcal | Carbohydrates: 41g | Protein: 5g | Fat: 8g | Sodium: 319mg | Fiber: 1g | Sugar: 10g

LOW FODMAP SUN-DRIED TOMATO PESTO

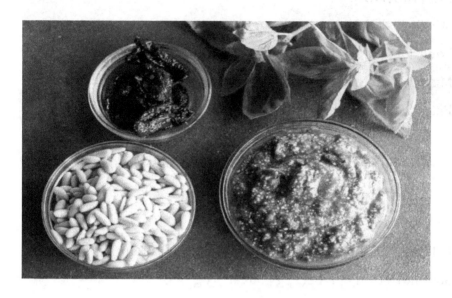

Makes: 8 Servings Prep Time: 10 minutes Total Time: 10 minutes

INGREDIENTS:

2 cups (16 g) fresh basil leaves

1 cup (100 g) grated Parmesan cheese

½ cup (76 g) lightly toasted European pine nuts, cooled

1 ¾- ounces (50 g) flexible sun-dried tomatoes

1 teaspoon kosher salt or to taste

1 cup (240 ml) Garlic-Infused Oil, made with olive oil, or purchased equivalent

PREPARATION:

Place basil, cheese, pine nuts, sun-dried tomatoes, and 1 teaspoon salt in a food processor fitted with a metal blade. Pulse on and off until finely chopped. Turn on the machine and add oil slowly and continue processing until a smooth paste is formed. Taste the mixture and add seasoning according to it. It is ready to use. You can refrigerate it for 2 weeks.

NUTRITION

Calories: 442kcal | Carbohydrates: 8g | Protein: 15g | Fat: 41g | Saturated Fat: 5g | Cholesterol: 26mg | Sodium: 455mg | Potassium: 211mg | Fiber: 2g | Sugar: 1g | Vitamin A: 3376IU | Vitamin C: 11mg | Calcium: 433mg | Iron: 2mg

LOW FODMAP MASALA CHAI

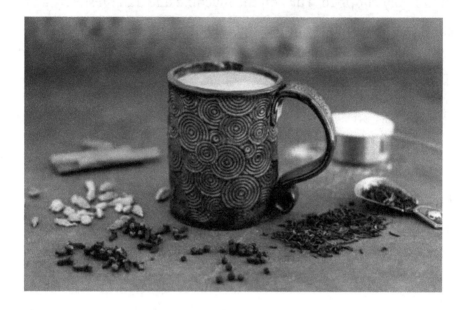

Makes: 2 Servings Prep Time: 2 minutes Cook Time: 6 minutes
Total Time: 8 minutes

INGREDIENTS:

1 ½ cups (360 ml) water

2 green cardamom pods

1 whole clove

1 whole black peppercorn

1/16 teaspoon ground cinnamon

Pinch ground ginger; optional

1/8- ounce (4 g) loose black tea, such as a hearty Assam

¼ cup to ½ cup (60 ml to 120 ml) lactose-free whole milk; or to taste

1 to 3 teaspoons sugar; or to taste

PREPARATION:

Put water in a pot and place it overheat. Add cardamoms along with peppercorn, clove, ground ginger, and cinnamon. Add your loose tea and cook for 3 minutes.

Add milk as much milky tea as you want and add some sugar to taste. Serve it immediately in cups.

NUTRITION

Calories: 42kcal | Carbohydrates: 7g | Protein: 2g | Fat: 1g | Saturated Fat: 1g | Sodium: 10mg | Potassium: 34mg | Fiber: 1g | Sugar: 4g | Vitamin C: 1mg | Calcium: 17mg | Iron: 1mg

VEGAN LOW FODMAP CRISP TOPPING

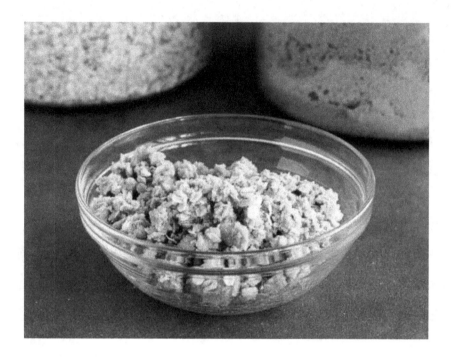

Makes: 8 Servings Prep Time: 10 minutes Total Time: 10 minutes

INGREDIENTS:

¾ cup (160 g) firmly packed light brown sugar

¾ cup (109 g) low FODMAP gluten-free flour, such as Bob's Red Mill Gluten Free 1 to 1 Baking Flour

¾ cup (74 g) old-fashioned rolled oats (not instant or quick oats); use gluten-free if following a gluten-free diet

¼ teaspoon cinnamon

¼ teaspoon salt

½ cup (120 ml) melted coconut oil, either refined or unrefined

PREPARATION:

Put sugar, oats, cinnamon, flour, and salt in a bowl and mix well. Add melted oil and stir until all mixture gets mixed. The crisp is ready to use.

NUTRITION

Calories: 268kcal | Carbohydrates: 35g | Protein: 2g | Fat: 15g | Sodium: 73mg | Fiber: 1g | Sugar: 18g

LOW FODMAP PEACHES AND CREAM POPSICLES WITH RASPBERRIES

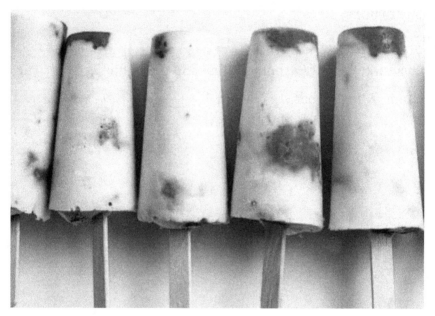

Makes: 8 Servings Prep Time: 15 minutes Freeze Time: 8 hours
Total Time: 8 hours 15 minutes

INGREDIENTS:

8 ½- ounces (240 g) chopped peaches, peeled stones discarded; buy 3 peaches to be safe

1 cup (245 g) thick vanilla lactose-free yogurt

1 tablespoon plus 1 teaspoon honey, divided

½ teaspoon lemon juice, divided

2 ¾- ounces (75 g) fresh raspberries

PREPARATION:

Chop peaches and add them to a blender along with lime juice, yogurt, and honey. Blend it well to form a smooth paste. Get ready the mold of your popsicles.

In a small bowl mash the raspberries with 1 teaspoon honey and the remaining ¼ teaspoon lemon juice. Spoon a small amount of the mashed raspberries into each pop mold.

Fill molds halfway with yogurt/peach mixture, add more berry purée. Top with more yogurt mixture. Insert wooden sticks that come with your popsicle set. Freeze it overnight and it is ready to eat.

NUTRITION

Calories: 49kcal | Carbohydrates: 10g | Protein: 2g | Fat: 1g | Sodium: 1mg | Fiber: 2g | Sugar: 7g | Vitamin C: 1mg

LOW FODMAP NO-CHURN VANILLA ICE CREAM WITH CHOCOLATE COVERED ALMONDS

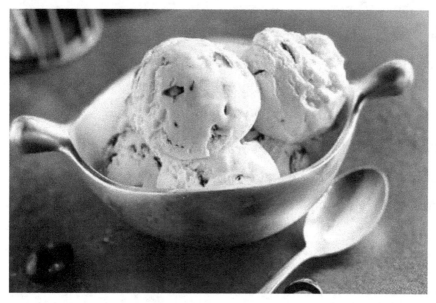

Makes: 10 Servings Prep Time: 15 minutes Dairy Resting Time & Chilling Time: 16 hours Total Time: 16 hours 15 minutes

INGREDIENTS:

2 cups (480 ml) lactose-free heavy cream, chilled

½ cup (99 g) sugar; use superfine if you have it

1 vanilla bean, split

1 tablespoon whiskey

Pinch salt

½ cup (90 g) dark chocolate covered almonds (about 22 nuts), chopped

PREPARATION:

Put chilled cream and sugar in a mixer. Add vanilla bean seeds into the mixture. Add a pinch of salt and whiskey. Beat it with an electric beater. After getting done fold it in chopped dark chocolate covered almonds. Put it in a container and freeze overnight.

NUTRITION

Calories: 251kcal | Carbohydrates: 17g | Protein: 1g | Fat: 12g | Sodium: 1mg | Sugar: 12g

LOW FODMAP NO-CHURN VANILLA ICE CREAM

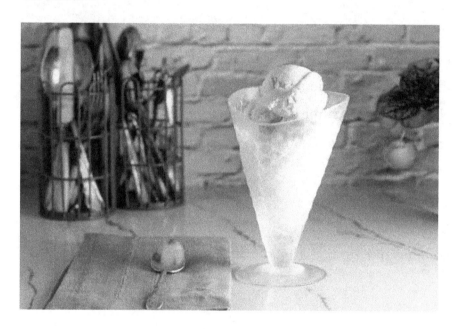

Makes: 10 Servings Prep Time: 15 minutes Dairy Resting Time & Chilling Time: 16 hours Total Time: 16 hours 15 minutes

INGREDIENTS:

2 cups (480 ml) lactose-free heavy cream, chilled

2 teaspoons vanilla extract

Pinch salt

1, 14- ounce (397 g) can lactose-free sweetened condensed milk

PREPARATION:

Mix chilled cream, vanilla, and salt in a large mixing bowl. Beat this mixture with an electric mixer Take care not to over-beat it.

Put it into an airtight container and freeze until firm, preferably overnight. Allow sitting for a few minutes at room temperature. Serve and enjoy immediately as it melts faster than conventional ice cream.

NUTRITION

Calories: 296kcal | Carbohydrates: 24g | Protein: 4g | Fat: 14g | Sodium: 1mg | Sugar: 1g

LOW FODMAP CANTALOUPE, CUCUMBER AND BURRATA SALAD

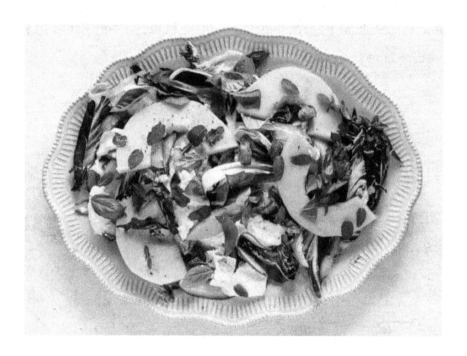

Makes: 8 Servings Prep Time: 15 minutes Total Time: 15 minutes

INGREDIENTS:

2- pounds (910 g) peeled, seeded, sliced ripe cantaloupe

Kosher salt

Freshly ground black pepper

1 small head (about 300 g) radicchio, cored and cut or torn into bite-sized pieces

3 Persian cucumbers, trimmed, sliced into wide, thin ribbons

8- ounces (225 g) burrata; typically about 2 pieces

Fresh basil leaves; a small handful

Fresh mint leaves; a small handful

Low FODMAP Red Wine Vinaigrette

PREPARATION:

Have a bowl or platter to set a salad. First of all place melon around the platter. Arrange radicchio over the melon. Now decorate the top with cucumbers.

Cut the burrata into a bite-sized piece and put it at the top so that liquid can be spilled over. Cut and tear herbs and spread over salad. You can refrigerate it and it is ready to serve.

NUTRITION

Calories: 129kcal | Carbohydrates: 15g | Protein: 6g | Fat: 7g | Saturated Fat: 1g | Sodium: 1mg | Potassium: 31mg | Fiber: 2g | Sugar: 13g | Vitamin A: 22IU | Vitamin C: 1mg | Calcium: 3mg | Iron: 1mg

LOW FODMAP CARROT-GINGER SOUP

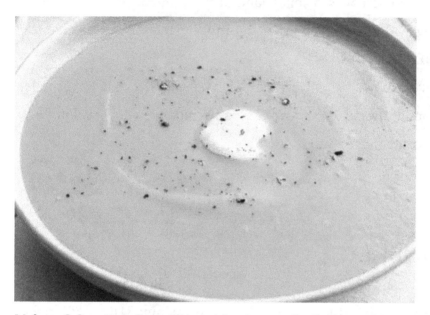

Makes: 8 Servings Prep Time: 10 minutes Cook Time: 30 minutes
Total Time: 40 minutes

INGREDIENTS:

1 teaspoon extra-virgin olive oil or butter

½ cup coarsely chopped fennel bulb

1 medium celery stalk, coarsely chopped

2 tablespoons grated peeled fresh ginger, plus more as needed

6 cups Nourishing Vegetable Broth, from the book or use our Low
FODMAP Vegetable Broth

6 medium carrots, peeled and coarsely chopped

2 medium yellow potatoes, coarsely chopped

¼ teaspoon freshly ground black pepper plus more as needed

¼ teaspoon salt plus more as needed (optional)

½ cup vegan yogurt, optional

PREPARATION:

In a large pot, heat the oil over medium-high heat. Add the fennel and celery, and sauté for 5 minutes, or until softened. Reduce the heat to medium. Add the ginger, and cook, stirring constantly, for 2 minutes.

Add carrots, pepper, potatoes, broth, and salt in a pot. Bring it to the boil. Cover and cook until potatoes get tender.

Using a food processor blend the soup mixture to form puree consistency. Taste and add seasonings according to your taste. Serve it immediately.

NUTRITION

Calories: 69kcal | Carbohydrates: 14g | Protein: 1g | Fat: 1g | Sodium: 73mg | Fiber: 2g | Sugar: 3g

LOW FODMAP TOFU SALAD

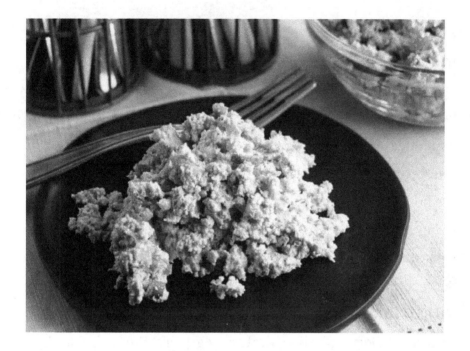

Makes: 6 Servings Prep Time: 5 minutes Freezing Time: 8 hours

Total Time: 8 hours 5 minutes

INGREDIENTS:

14- ounce (400 g) container of the firm or extra-firm tofu in water

½ cup (113 g) mayonnaise

2 teaspoons Dijon mustard

2 teaspoons lemon juice

1 medium carrot, peeled and shredded

1 medium stalk celery, finely diced

2 tablespoons chopped scallions, green parts only

Kosher salt

Freshly ground black pepper

Dulse flakes; optional

PREPARATION:

Put tofu in the freezer overnight. Take it out and crumble it. Press tofu to take out as much water as you can.

Put tofu in a mixing bowl and add mustard, lemon juice, mayonnaise, carrot, scallion greens, and celery. Mix it and taste it according to your taste. It is ready to serve.

NUTRITION

Calories: 206kcal | Carbohydrates: 3g | Protein: 7g | Fat: 18g | Saturated Fat: 2g | Cholesterol: 8mg | Sodium: 144mg | Fiber: 1g | Sugar: 1g | Vitamin A: 13IU | Vitamin C: 1mg | Iron: 1mg

LOW FODMAP ORANGE CARROT JUICE

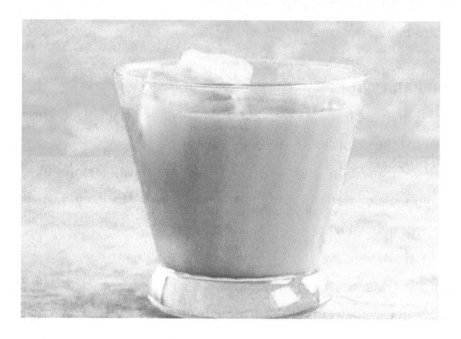

Makes: 2 Servings Prep Time: 5 minutes Total Time: 5 minutes

INGREDIENTS:

Basic Blend:

½ cup (120 ml) freshly squeezed carrot juice

½ cup (120 ml) freshly squeezed orange juice

Add-Ons:

¼ cup (60 ml) UHT unsweetened coconut milk

2 tablespoons low FODMAP whey protein isolate, such as Opportunities Grass-Fed Whey Protein Isolate

Ice

PREPARATION:

1st version: combine carrot and orange juice and mix them well. The juice is ready to drink.

2nd version: coconut milk can be added in the 1st version. Mix well or put them in a mixer.

3rd version: Place carrot juice, orange juice, coconut milk, protein powder, and ice in a blender and zap it until frothy, icy, and blended. Serve immediately.

NUTRITION

Calories: 79kcal | Carbohydrates: 10g | Protein: 8g | Fat: 1g

LOW FODMAP CREAM OF TOMATO SOUP WITH GRILLED CHEESE CROUTONS

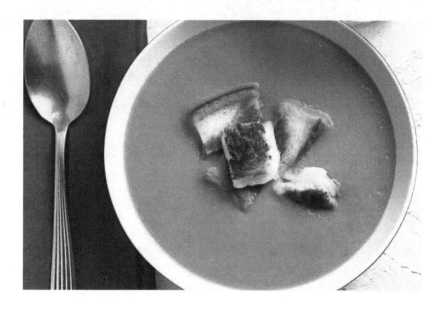

Makes: 3 Servings Prep Time: 15 minutes Cook Time: 25 minutes

Total Time: 40 minutes

At room temperature, sliced very thinly

PREPARATION:

For the Soup: Heat oil over low-medium heat in a large Dutch oven or heavy pot until shimmering. Add scallion greens and sauté until softened but not browned.

Add tomatoes and juice and crush tomatoes with a masher. Add seasonings and bring to a boil.

Adjust heat to a simmer, cover pot, and cook for 15 minutes. Taste and adjust seasoning.

Carefully transfer to blender and purée, or purée right in the pot if you have an immersion blender. You can leave as is, or for a more classic texture, strain through a fine-meshed strainer and return to pot to reheat. Add cream, heat gently, but do not boil. Keep warm.

For the Grilled Cheese Croutons: You make the grilled cheese while the soup is cooking to save time if you want to multitask.

Lay your bread out on your work surface in front of you and spread a tablespoon of mayonnaise on each slice, edge to edge, covering completely.

Place a large nonstick or cast-iron pan on the stove over low heat and add butter. Melt the butter and swirl it around the pan. Place two slices of bread in the pan, mayo side down. Divide cheese between the two pieces of bread and top with remaining bread, mayo side up. Increase heat to low-medium. Cook until the bottom is golden brown, flip, and continue cooking until the second side is equally crispy and golden and cheese is melted.

Pour hot soup into warm bowls. Cut sandwiches into small square "croutons", about 1-inch (2.5 cm) across. Divide croutons amongst bowls and serve immediately.

NUTRITION

Calories: 524kcal | Carbohydrates: 48g | Protein: 13g | Fat: 47g |
Saturated Fat: 2g | Cholesterol: 8mg | Sodium: 744mg | Sugar: 14g

LOW FODMAP CARAMELIZED PINEAPPLE SAUCE

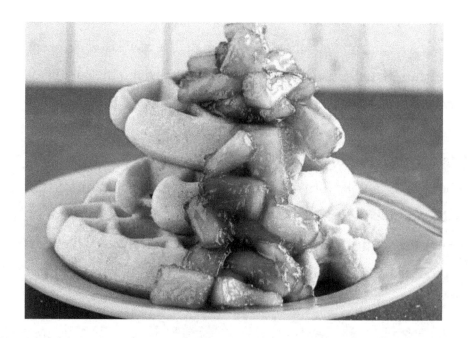

Makes: 8 Servings Prep Time: 5 minutes Cook Time: 10 minutes
Total Time: 15 minutes

INGREDIENTS:

6 tablespoons (85 g) unsalted butter, cut into pieces

½ cup (107 g) firmly packed light brown sugar

4 cups (560 g) fresh pineapple chunks

¾ cup (180 ml) pure maple syrup

PREPARATION:

Put butter in a pot and melt it. Add brown sugar and cook until sugar gets dissolved. Add pineapples and cook until butter/sugar mixture gets caramelize and toss pineapple well. Add maple syrup and cook all get mixed well. Remove from heat and let it cool. It is ready to eat now.

NUTRITION

Calories: 189kcal | Carbohydrates: 29g | Protein: 1g | Fat: 8g | Sodium: 2mg | Potassium: 50mg | Fiber: 1g | Sugar: 13g | Calcium: 24mg | Iron: 1mg

LOW FODMAP RANCH DRESSING

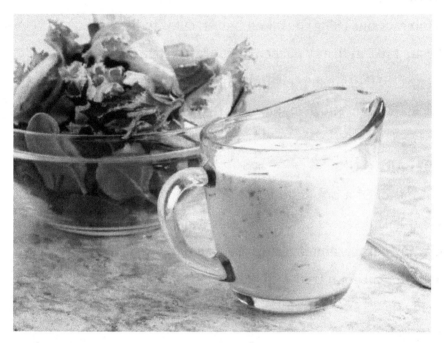

Makes: 4 Servings Prep Time: 10 minutes Total Time: 10 minutes

INGREDIENTS:

½ cup (120 ml) lactose-free whole milk

2 teaspoons freshly squeezed lemon juice

½ cup (113 g) mayonnaise

2 tablespoons finely chopped fresh chives or 2 teaspoons dried chives

1 tablespoon finely chopped fresh dill or 1 teaspoon dried dill

1 tablespoon finely chopped fresh flat-leaf parsley or 1 teaspoon dried parsley

1 tablespoon finely chopped scallions, green parts only

2 teaspoons Garlic-Infused Oil, made with vegetable oil or purchased garlic-flavored vegetable oil

½ teaspoon Dijon mustard

Kosher salt

Freshly ground black pepper

PREPARATION:

Mix lime juice and milk in a jar and let it set aside until it gets thick. Add mayonnaise, scallions, chives, parsley, dill, oil, and mustard. Cover it and shake it well. Add seasonings according to taste. The dressing is ready to use.

NUTRITION

Calories: 235kcal | Carbohydrates: 2g | Protein: 1g | Fat: 25g | Saturated Fat: 3g | Cholesterol: 12mg | Sodium: 195mg | Fiber: 1g | Sugar: 2g | Vitamin A: 19IU | Iron: 1mg

LOW FODMAP PASTA PRIMAVERA

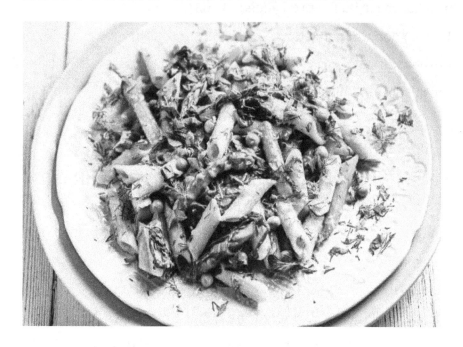

Makes: 6 Servings Prep Time: 10 minutes Cook Time: 15 minutes
Total Time: 25 minutes

INGREDIENTS:

2 tablespoons Onion-Infused Oil, made with shallots and olive oil;
extra if needed

1/3 cup (24 g) chopped chives or scallion greens

3 ½ cups (840 ml) water

Kosher salt

12- ounces (340 g) low FODMAP, gluten-free penne, such as Jovial
brand

3 asparagus stalks, trimmed, cut into 2-inch (5 cm) lengths

3- ounces (85 g) fresh baby arugula leaves

3- ounces (85 g) fresh baby spinach leaves

60 grams frozen peas, about 1/3 cup

2 tablespoons unsalted butter

3- ounces (85 g) finely grated Parmesan cheese

2 tablespoons freshly squeezed lemon juice, plus 1 teaspoon finely grated lemon zest

2 tablespoons chopped fresh dill

2 tablespoons chopped fresh tarragon

Freshly ground black pepper

PREPARATION:

Add oil to a pan and heat it. Add scallion green until they get soft and brown. Add pasta, water, and a pinch of salt. Stir well and bring it to a boil. After 4 minutes add the asparagus and cook for about 30 seconds, then stir the arugula and spinach into the pasta and water. Re-cover the pot. Keep cooking until pasta gets tender. Do not let water vanished. Add peas and cook for 30 seconds. Remove from heat and add lemon zest, lime juice, and parmesan and stir well. It is ready to use.

NUTRITION

Calories: 325kcal | Carbohydrates: 44g | Protein: 10g | Fat: 13g | Sodium: 139mg | Fiber: 2g | Calcium: 4mg

LOW FODMAP GRATED CARROT SALAD

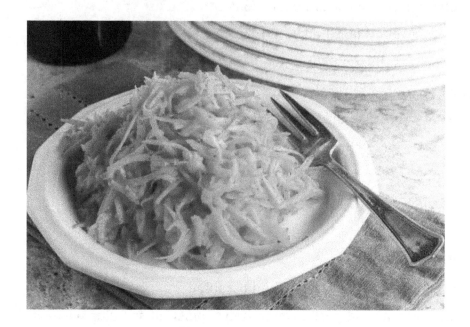

Makes: 6 Servings Prep Time: 10 minutes Total Time: 10 minutes

INGREDIENTS:

1- Pound (455 g) carrots, trimmed and peeled, shredded

1 fresh large heavy lemon, halved, pitted

2 to 4 tablespoons (2 tablespoons to 60 ml) extra-virgin olive oil, divided

Kosher salt

Freshly ground black pepper

PREPARATION:

Peel and grate carrots. Add a little amount of oil and lime juice and toss well. Add seasonings according to your taste. Mix well and you are set to eat.

NUTRITION

Calories: 73kcal | Carbohydrates: 7g | Protein: 1g | Fat: 5g | Saturated Fat: 1g | Sodium: 1mg | Fiber: 2g | Sugar: 3g

NO FODMAP FRUIT SALAD

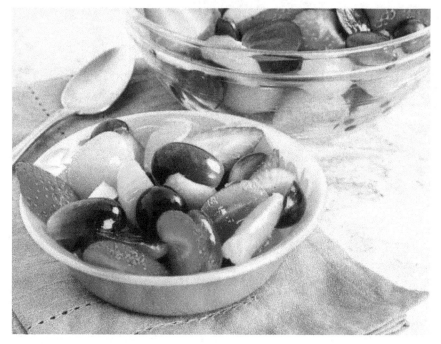

Makes: 6 Servings Prep Time: 10 minutes Total Time: 10 minutes

INGREDIENTS:

1- Pound (455 g) strawberries

4 clementines; (or 2 navel oranges)

2 cups (300 g) grapes; I like a mixture of seedless black, green and red

PREPARATION:

Hull the strawberries, then halve or quarter. Peel and section the clementines. Halve the grapes.

Just mix all fruits well and your fruit salad is ready to eat.

NUTRITION

Calories: 102kcal | Carbohydrates: 26g | Protein: 1g | Fat: 1g | Saturated Fat: 1g | Sodium: 3mg | Potassium: 354mg | Fiber: 3g | Sugar: 20g | Vitamin A: 61IU | Vitamin C: 71mg | Calcium: 35mg | Iron: 1mg

---

NO FODMAP MALT VINEGAR SALAD DRESSING

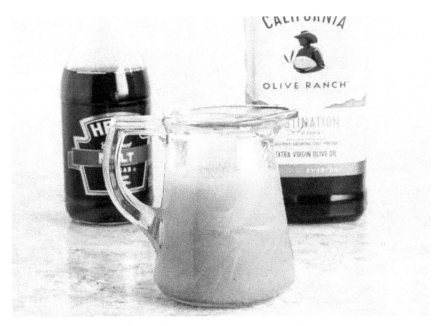

Makes: 8 Servings Prep Time: 5 minutes Total Time: 5 minutes

INGREDIENTS:

¾ cup (180 ml) extra virgin olive oil

1/3 cup (75 ml) malt vinegar

Kosher salt

Freshly ground black pepper

PREPARATION:

Mix and shake vinegar and oil together in a jar. Add salt and pepper according to taste and mix well. The dressing is ready to use or you can place it in a refrigerator.

NUTRITION

Calories: 198kcal | Carbohydrates: 1g | Fat: 22g | Saturated Fat: 3g | Sodium: 1mg | Sugar: 1g | Iron: 1mg

NO FODMAP VEGETABLE SALAD

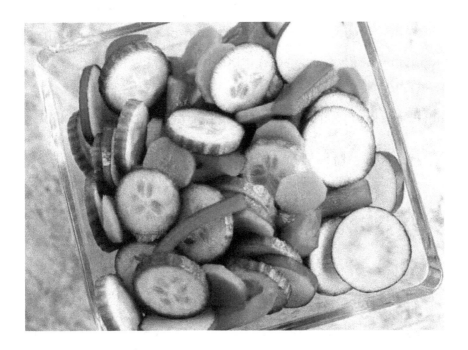

Makes: 4 Servings Prep Time: 5 minutes Total Time: 5 minutes

INGREDIENTS:

6 red radishes, trimmed, sliced crosswise into discs

2 medium carrots, trimmed, peeled, and cut crosswise into discs

2 small Persian cucumbers or half an English hothouse cucumber, cut crosswise into discs

1 red bell pepper, cored and cut into strips

Kosher salt; optional

Freshly ground black pepper; optional

Olive oil; optional

No FODMAP Malt Vinegar Salad Dressing

PREPARATION:

Simply toss the vegetables together and the salad is ready to enjoy. Add seasonings including salt and pepper in the required amount and enjoy the salad. A little vinegar can be added.

NUTRITION

Calories: 32kcal | Carbohydrates: 6g | Protein: 1g | Fat: 1g | Fiber: 2g | Sugar: 3g

---

LOW FODMAP EGGPLANT DIP

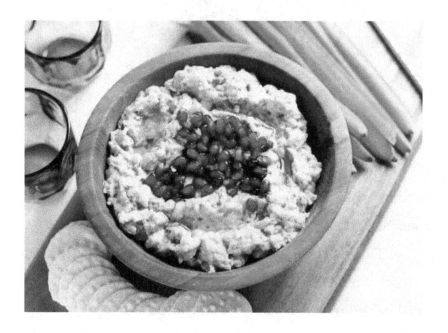

Makes: 8 Servings Prep Time: 10 minutes Cook Time: 1 hour Total Time: 1 hour 10 minutes

INGREDIENTS:

2, large globe eggplants, about 1 ½ pounds/680 g each, washed and dried

¼ cup (60 ml) tahini

1 tablespoon freshly squeezed lemon juice, or to taste

Kosher salt

Garlic-Infused Olive Oil

Pomegranate seeds; optional

PREPARATION:

Position rack in the upper part of the oven. Preheat oven to 400°F (200°C). Place eggplant directly on the rack (or on a rimmed baking sheet if you want to prevent any potential drips in your oven) and roast for about an hour or until the eggplant is super soft, tender, and wrinkly. Remove and cool.

Peel eggplant and take out the flesh. Mash the flesh in a bowl or make a puree by blending it in a blender. Add tahini and lemon juice according to taste. Taste and add salt and pepper according to need. Take it in a bowl. Add oil and garnish it with pomegranate seeds. It is all set to use.

NUTRITION

Calories: 78kcal | Carbohydrates: 10g | Protein: 3g | Fat: 4g | Saturated Fat: 1g | Sodium: 3mg | Potassium: 34mg | Fiber: 5g | Sugar: 3g | Vitamin C: 1mg | Calcium: 10mg | Iron: 1mg

LOW FODMAP CARROT CONSOMMÉ

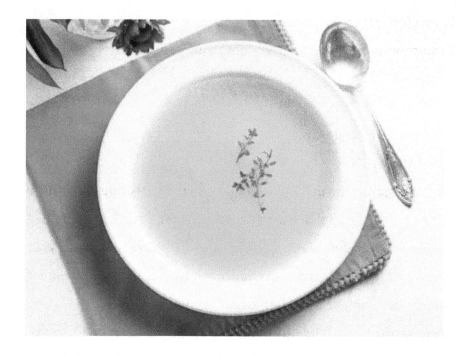

Makes: 8 Servings Prep Time: 10 minutes Cook Time: 3 hours

Total Time: 3 hours 10 minutes

INGREDIENTS:

3 quarts (2.8 L) water

4- pounds (1.8 kg) carrots, trimmed, peeled, and cut into large chunks

1 cup (72 g) chopped leeks, green parts only

2- Inches (5 cm) fresh ginger, peeled and cut in half lengthwise

5 black peppercorns

2 whole cloves

2 bay leaves

2 sprigs fresh thyme

1 celery stalk, trimmed and cut into large chunks

Kosher salt

PREPARATION:

Add all vegetables in water to a pot. Cook them on high heat and then simmer them for 3 hours. After getting done, pass it on a strainer and discard the vegetables. Taste the consomme and add seasonings. Heat it before serving.

NUTRITION

Calories: 97kcal | Carbohydrates: 23g | Protein: 3g | Fat: 1g | Saturated Fat: 1g | Sodium: 18mg | Fiber: 7g | Sugar: 11g | Calcium: 11mg

EASY STOVETOP LOW FODMAP MAC AND CHEESE

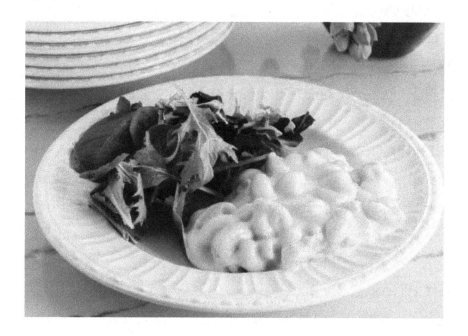

Makes: 6 Servings Prep Time: 10 minutes Cook Time: 15 minutes Total Time: 25 minutes

INGREDIENTS:

12- ounces (340 g) low FODMAP, gluten-free elbow pasta, such as Jovial brand

½ cup (1 stick; 113 g) unsalted butter, cut into pieces

½ cup (73 g) low FODMAP, gluten-free all-purpose flour

1 ¼ teaspoon dry, powdered mustard

1 teaspoon kosher salt

½ teaspoon white pepper

3 cups (720 ml) lactose-free whole milk, at room temperature

8- ounces (225 g) sharp cheddar cheese, shredded; I like using orange colored

PREPARATION:

Bring a large pot with salted water and bring to a boil and cook the pasta till al dente; do not over-cook. Drain and set aside.

Simultaneously, take another pot and add butter to it. Heat it and melt it. Add flour, salt, mustard, and pepper. Cook it for 1 to 2 minutes. Gradually add milk and cook until the sauce gets thickened. Remove from heat and add pasta and fold it well. Serve it.

NUTRITION

Calories: 601kcal | Carbohydrates: 58g | Protein: 19g | Fat: 33g | Saturated Fat: 1g | Sodium: 619mg | Fiber: 2g | Sugar: 6g

LOW FODMAP JAPANESE PICKLES

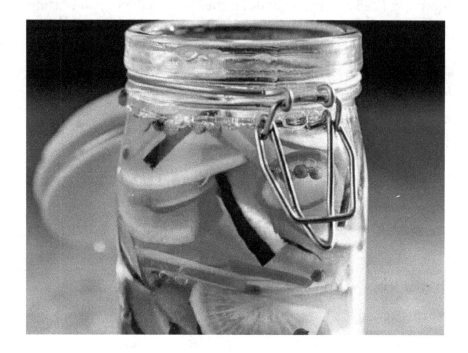

Makes: 6 Servings Prep Time: 5 minutes Cook Time: 2 minutes
Cooking Time: 30 minutes Total Time: 37 minutes

INGREDIENTS:

Pickling Liquor:

1 teaspoon cilantro seeds

1 teaspoon cumin seeds

¼ cup (60 ml) water

Juice of 1 lime

1 to 2 tablespoons caster sugar

1 teaspoon of sea salt

Vegetables:

½ standard cucumber finely sliced, seeds removed

3- Ounces (55 g) daikon, finely sliced

2- Ounces (55 g) salad radishes, finely sliced

½ cup (120 ml) rice or white vinegar

PREPARATION:

Place a non-stick pan over heat and add cilantro and cumin seeds and cook for 1 to 2 minutes.

Add all remaining pickle ingredients and cook. Once the sugar and salt get dissolved remove the pan from heat. Let it cool. Add vegetables and vinegar and let it pickle. Store it in an airtight jar.

NUTRITION

Calories: 29kcal | Carbohydrates: 6g | Protein: 1g | Fat: 1g | Saturated Fat: 1g | Sodium: 392mg | Potassium: 6mg | Fiber: 1g | Sugar: 4g | Calcium: 3mg | Iron: 1mg

LOW FODMAP LEMON GRANITA

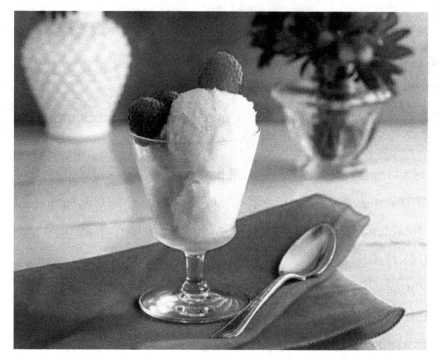

Makes: 8 Servings Prep Time: 15 minutes Cook Time: 3 minutes

Chilling Time: 4 hours Total Time: 4 hours 18 minutes

INGREDIENTS:

2 ½ cups (600 ml) water, divided

1 cup (198 g) sugar

1 cup (240 ml) freshly squeezed lemon juice

1 ½ teaspoon finely grated lemon zest

Optional: pomegranate seeds, or fresh firm raspberries

PREPARATION:

Combine half of the water and sugar in a medium saucepan. Stir to wet the sugar. Place over medium heat and bring to a simmer. Cook until the sugar dissolves, swirling the pot once or twice. Remove from the heat, cool to room temperature, and stir in the remaining water, lemon juice, and zest. Pour into an 8-inch (20 cm) or 9-inch (23 cm) metal pan.

Freeze for 45 minutes or until it starts getting freeze. Take a fork and take out the frozen parts other than the liquid part. Check again and again and take out all of the crystals. This granita is ready to use.

NUTRITION

Calories: 122kcal | Carbohydrates: 32g | Protein: 1g | Sodium: 4mg | Fiber: 1g | Sugar: 30g | Calcium: 2mg

CPSIA information can be obtained
at www.ICGtesting.com
Printed in the USA
BVHW092105240621
610373BV00002B/286